REIKI:

An Ancient Healing Art Revisited

Marguerite Antonio

iUniverse, Inc.
Bloomington

Reiki: An Ancient Healing Art Revisited

iUniverse books may be ordered through booksellers or by contacting:

iUniverse
1663 Liberty Drive
Bloomington, IN 47403
www.iuniverse.com
1-800-Authors (1-800-288-4677)

ISBN: 978-1-4502-8482-0 (pbk)
ISBN: 978-1-4502-8484-4 (cloth)
ISBN: 978-1-4502-8483-7 (ebk)

Library of Congress Control Number: 2010919512

Printed in the United States of America

iUniverse rev. date: 3/22/11

— Contents —

— Preface —

Why a Book about Reiki?

I wrote this book for those who are interested in learning more about the ancient healing art of Reiki. It reflects my experience as a Reiki practitioner and is founded in the traditional Usui System. However, modern science has learned much regarding "subtle energies" since the time Dr. Usui first set down the precepts of Reiki therapy, and I discuss some of these findings in these pages.

I have been involved with healing arts for more than twenty years. I am a reflexologist certified with the Canadian Reflexology Association, a Usui Reiki Master Teacher certified with the Canadian Reiki Association, and a certified Karuna Reiki Master. I have also studied and have certification in the healing modalities of herbalism, bio-energy nutrition, and ear candling. I use Reiki both in conjunction with these other modalities and alone in my practice. Invariably, my clients are more relaxed and feel better after a treatment. Several years ago, I was asked to teach Reiki, but I found that there simply wasn't sufficient written information available to give my students. Much of what I have learned was taught to me orally and in practice with my own Reiki Master. I decided to write and self publish a text for my Reiki classes.

Please Note: This text is written for your interest only and is not meant to take the place of personal instruction and attunement from a qualified Reiki Master. Only a Reiki Master can help you capture the essence of real Reiki energy, without which you cannot be a qualified Reiki practitioner. I have provided websites and an e-mail address at the back of the book to help you locate a master near you.

Becoming a Healer

The journey to becoming a natural healer is indeed that—a journey. This journey is ongoing and encompasses all aspects of your life: mental, emotional, physical, and spiritual. If you are reading this book or have gone to a healing seminar, you are already on the path.

I have identified five stages in the process of becoming a natural healing practitioner. These stages may happen in any order and at any time of your life. Each of us comes to this place and this time in our own way through our own life plan. These stages of learning are well documented in books written on various healing modalities, from ancient writings to the more modern New Age texts. These stages are as follows:

1. Inheritance
2. The Calling
3. The Quest
4. Apprenticeship
5. Practicing the Art of Healing

Inheritance

I believe that anyone can learn the techniques of natural healing, be it shamanism, native healing, reflexology, herbalism, faith healing, acupuncture, or Reiki. Many of us combine several of these techniques in our practice quite successfully. What I speak of here is the potential for and/or predilection toward helping others and our own unique personal and familial history of doing so. By looking at your own history in respect to this subject, you will find the links. I was brought up in the southern Alberta Bible Belt. One of my grandparents was a church leader and healer in his day, and my grandmother on the other side of the family lived to age of 106. She often used plain old remedies to help heal the ills within my family—such as chicken soup for colds and flu, lavender for relaxation, and mustard poultices for coughs—combined with lots of TLC. Later, when I studied herbalism, I came to appreciate the wisdom of her healing practices.

I also fully appreciate my Christian heritage, for it taught me how to connect with God and grow in spirit. Healing work involves the spiritual aspect of life, as well as the physical, emotional, and mental. However, I must emphasize that while many natural healing arts involve working with spirit, they are not religions themselves or even religious in nature. A person's religious heritage or lack thereof has no bearing on his or her ability to heal or be healed. Still, practitioners and those they seek to heal are undoubtedly influenced by their unique heritage and spiritual lessons.

Look at your own history. You will see a pattern emerge!

The Calling

Like me, you may have known that you wanted to be a healer from a very young age as you tried to rescue wounded birdies or injured animals and pleaded with your parents to help you save them. Or you may have had a life-altering experience that guided you to become a healer. This feeling or desire is often enhanced by recurring dreams or daydreams that just won't go away and a "coincidence" that isn't really as random as you first thought.

Along with the calling, there is an experience that further pushes you into the realm of natural healing. It may have been a severe illness, a near-death experience for yourself or a loved one, an accidental purchase of a book, or being involved in a seminar that just made it click for you, that left you with the profound desire to do more and learn more about a certain healing modality.

The Quest

The calling then leads you to a desire to learn more, experience more, and open up to spirituality in new ways. It encourages you to find answers. This is the point at which you should find a teacher, a guide, or a process by which to help fulfill your longing and desire to learn.

Apprenticeship

An apprenticeship can take a few different forms. You may choose to spend time with elders who are wiser and more learned than you. You may enroll in a school program that offers what you need and desire. Or you may choose to begin your own individual study through books, seminars, and deep meditation or prayer to connect you more securely with your own spirit guides and mentors. For many of us, apprenticeship is often all of these things.

Practicing the Art of Healing

When your mentors or teachers deem you to have learned the essentials of the healing modality or healing art of your choice, you are ready to set up a practice and ply your trade.

In natural healing, learning is ongoing and ever-enlightening.

Reiki Defined

Reiki (pronounced *ray-key*) is a very ancient healing art that was revived by Dr. M. Usui in Japan just before the Second World War. Its origin may have been Tibetan, Indian, or Egyptian, as historical evidence shows peoples from all of these areas used Reiki as a tool for healing and well-being well before the time of Christ. The Japanese character of Rei means spiritual wisdom and the Ki denotes life-force energy. Life-force energy is essential to all that we do. It animates the human body on a cellular level and is the prime source of our thoughts and ideas. Reiki works at the physical as well as the emotional, mental, and spiritual levels to enhance this energy.

A Reiki treatment is a deeply relaxing experience that:

- Promotes relaxation on a mental, physical, and spiritual level
- Balances and enhances body energy
- Encourages the release of disease on all levels
- Enhances the body's innate ability to heal by having a positive effect on the endocrine and immune system.
- Is a deeply relaxing experience that helps trigger the parasympathetic nervous system, which sustains all the body's functions and awakens the body's

own ability to self-heal and restore balance. Reiki's spiritually guided life-force energy also assists the parasympathetic system in its function. This system nurtures and nourishes the body and is responsible for rejuvenating and regenerating all the cells of the body.

Anyone committed to the healing of oneself and others can learn to do Reiki. Reiki is, as yet, not taught in schools or colleges but is passed down directly from the Reiki Master to the student in workshops or seminars. This way, the students learn to focus this loving, healing energy through their palms, as well as how to awaken this latent but natural talent within themselves.

Reiki is *not*:

- A cure-all
- A cult or religious belief
- Invasive or harmful to the receiver or giver in any way
- Applicable for only a select few; anyone can learn (or relearn) this healing art.

A Brief History of Reiki

Reiki is a very ancient healing art that is believed to have been practiced by monks in Tibet, Egypt, and India for thousands of years. There are several books and many theories about how this ancient art was revived by a Dr. Mikao Usui in Japan prior to World War II. Unfortunately, much of Dr. Usui's documentation on Reiki and how he came to use it was lost during the war, so there doesn't seem to be a definitive history.

Some say Dr. Usui was a teacher in a Christian school in Japan; others say he was a Buddhist monk. What we do know for sure is that at some point, he became very intrigued by what we now call hands-on healing. He traveled to many monasteries and universities (some say even to the United States) over a period years to learn and observe healing forms and techniques. During this time of study and research, Dr. Usui found ancient Sanskrit writings in one of the older monasteries that were believed to be from ancient Tibet. He studied these writings in depth and came to the realization that further knowledge could only be acquired through deep meditation. It is said that in the spring of 1922, Dr. Usui went to a secluded area in the mountains north of Kyoto, Japan, where he fasted and meditated for twenty-one days. On the twentieth day, he saw a huge ball of light on the horizon. The ball of light sped toward him, but instead turning away from it, he embraced this energy and light and was taken on a mystical journey. He was shown a bubble of all the colors of the rainbow. Within this bubble were symbols that corresponded to the same Tibetan symbols in the Sanskrit writings he had been studying.

Dr. Usui came down from the mountain and began to heal himself and others using the symbols he had learned. Wanting to share the marvelous gift he had been given with as many of the needy as possible, he worked in the ghettos of Tokyo. He helped heal the sick and infirm and sent some to local priests who found them employment and means to earn a decent living. Soon, however, he found some familiar faces reentering his clinics. Puzzled, he questioned them and found that many had not valued the gift of healing and the new life he had offered, preferring instead the familiarity of the squalor in which they had lived. Disillusioned, Dr. Usui returned to the monasteries and eventually came to understand that he needed to teach gratitude along with the healing. After further study, reflection, and planning, he set down precepts based upon those ancient Sanskrit writings and his own experiences. These precepts would become the foundation for Reiki in the Usui system as we practice it today.

Though much was lost during World War II, the concept of Reiki as taught by Dr. Usui was passed on to Dr. Chujiro Hayashi. Dr. Hayashi continued in the original Usui Reiki tradition at his clinic in Tokyo, training others this healing art, and in 1935 agreed to accept a student from Hawaii. After several years of study with Dr. Hayashi, Mrs. Hawayo Takata took her knowledge back to Hawaii and set up a healing and training center there. She was a powerful healer, and over the next forty years, Mrs. Takata proceeded to train twenty-two students in the Reiki traditions and techniques until they too were initiated as Reiki Masters.

Most of the Reiki Masters practicing and teaching in North America today were trained by students of the original twenty-two masters who trained with Mrs. Takata in Hawaii.

This is just a brief summary of the history of Reiki. There are many books with more detailed accounts in libraries and reputable bookstores as well as on the Web at www. Reiki.org and www.reiki.ca.

How Reiki Is Taught

When teaching students this healing art, Dr. Usui implemented the teaching methods passed on by the ancients. He formulated precepts and concepts to help instill in his students not only that which is required to perform a healing treatment, but also the means by which a student could develop spiritually. His own experience taught him that technique alone would not instill the essence of Reiki. His Reiki Ideals are a method by which a student can recognize and act with greater spiritual awareness in his or her life.

The Reiki Ideals

Just for today, I will let go of anger.

Just for today, I will let go of worry.

Just for today, I will give thanks for my many blessings.

Just for today, I will do my work honestly.

Just for today, I will be kind to my neighbour and every living thing.

Reiki is taught in progressive levels by a Reiki Master. As the student learns the necessary elements of one level, he or she will receive a sacred symbol and its accompanying word or phrase (mantra). These symbols are derived from the ancient writings from which Dr. Usui gained the healing power and knowledge of Reiki. The words or phrases connected to them are simple mantras that depict the meaning and power of the symbols. Dr. Usui (and those teaching Reiki in the original format set out by him) believed that these symbols and mantras are to be memorized and held as sacred by the student. They are used by the healer to draw in and utilize the spirit-guided universal life-force energy. Each symbol has a specific meaning and application. To further enhance the flow of healing energy, the student undergoes an attunement. During the attunement ritual, the Reiki Master, following the example and teachings of Dr. Usui, embeds within the student the energies and attributes of the specific symbol the student was given. Without an attunement by a Reiki Master, a student, no matter how learned, is not receiving the full benefits of Reiki and is not able to pass on the full benefits to his or her clients or himself or herself. Learning the method for a Reiki treatment is important, but memorizing the symbols and their meanings and getting an attunement by a Reiki Master are essential to the practice of the art of Reiki.

There are now many forms and systems for using Reiki that have evolved from the original methodology in practice today. In this text, I have tried to remain as true to the original as possible, with a few added bits of information that science has now given us that prove the original theories.

— 1 —

Reiki Level One

The first level of Reiki taught to a student involves working with healing energy on the physical plane.

Subtle Energy

Human beings are more than what we appear to be. There is an invisible world that exists around and within us. It seems that more and more people have become more aware of this fact. For example:

- Discussions about this type of energy now tend to cause less eye rolling than they did a few years ago. We may not know what causes gravity, but we trust it to bring back the ball we toss into the air. We may not understand how air currents work, but we trust them to hold the plane we are in aloft as we fly.
- We are beginning to see what the ancients saw very clearly about subtle energies and healing—illness is a physical expression of inner discord that can be dealt with on the subtle plane. We who are interested in natural healing feel these energies

thrum through and around us, and science today is starting to recognize this too.

- Semyon Kirlian (a Russian doctor) first photographed these etheric patterns and auras around living things in 1940.
- Barbara Brennen (a NASA scientist) studied this energy and correlated her findings in a book called *Hands of Light*.
- As a result of the work of Delores Krieger, RN, nurses are studying and using Healing Touch in the hospital setting, and Reiki is often used in hospices to help ease the dying.
- Our ancient ancestors were well aware of the spirit/mind/body connection and left us a wonderful legacy of many differing but aligned techniques to assist us in the healing process. For instance, many Aboriginal peoples used the healing circle, ancient Egyptians were familiar with reflexology, and ancient Tibetans used Reiki. Humans are now starting to relearn these arts and utilize them as a means for healing and renewal both personally and in settings like alternative healing clinics and spas.

Energy Zones

Energy flows along the ten zones of the body. These are zones or meridians by which energy is transmitted. The chakras are portals, or energy centers, within these zones.

There are more than three hundred chakras, or energy centers. When using Reiki, the palms, feet, and seven main chakras are the ones that are given particular attention.

MAJOR CHAKRAS

Crown – 7

Brow – 6

Throat – 5

Heart – 4

Solar Plexus – 3

Sacral – 2

Base – 1

Palm

Foot

The Human Energy Field and Chakras

In the practice of Reiki, it is not essential that you be able to see auras or energy fields, but it is helpful to understand that life-force energy flows through the body (and all living matter) in lines or meridians to nurture every cell in that body. Think of chakras as energy gateways into and out of the body. There are some 360 such gateways throughout the body. They range in size and function, from the seven major chakras spaced along the spinal column to smaller ones in the hands, feet, behind the knees, and at the elbows, and even smaller ones scattered about the body for various functions. One of the major functions of the chakra network is to convey life-force energy to the nucleus of every living cell. Each chakra vibrates favorably to and can be seen in the aura (by those who see auras) as related to a specific color and is related to specific areas of the body. It is believed that Reiki helps to enhance the energy of the chakras, opening, cleansing, and ridding them of negativity, thus allowing the freer flow of energy through these essential gateways to the areas of the body to which they are aligned.

Palm:

- transmits healing energy

Sole of the feet:

- absorbs energy from the earth (planet)
- is involved in grounding of certain energies and helping to complete the circuit of healing energies

1. Base or Root:
    - located at the base of the spine and is our link to Earth and the planet
    - deals with all issues of the physical nature, such as the body, the senses and sensuality, sexuality, survival, aggression, and self-defense mechanisms
    - linked to the endocrine glands but also effects pelvis, hips, legs, and feet
    - vibrates to the color red
2. Sacral:
    - lies opposite to the sacral bone in the spine, between the navel and base (root)
    - deals with all issues of creativity and sexuality (the expression of)
    - the seat of joy, where the "inner child" naturally resides

- linked to testes in the male and ovaries in the female
- affects womb, kidneys, lower digestive tract, and lower back
- vibrates to the color orange

3. Solar Plexus:
    - located across the solar plexus where the feeling of "butterflies in the stomach" manifests
    - deals with the mind and personal means of expression, where lower emotions of fear, anxiety, insecurity, jealousy, and anger generate
    - creates an important link between mind and emotions, as negative energies related to thought and feels are processed here
    - the place where the "wounded child" dwells
    - affects solar and splenic nerve plexus, digestive system, pancreas, liver, gallbladder, diaphragm, and middle back
    - vibrates to the color yellow
4. Heart:
    - at the center of the chest
    - deals with the soul, inner guidance, and is the seat of the higher emotions based on unconditional love, empathy, compassion, true love, and friendship
    - linked to the thymus gland, affects cardiac and pulmonary nerve plexus, lungs heart, bronchia, chest, upper back, and arms

- vibrates to the color green (or pink when you are in love)

5. Throat:
    - found at the base of the neck and throat area
    - deals with communication and expression whether through speech, art, music, or dance. Involves truth and true expression of the soul
    - linked to thyroid and parathyroid glands
    - affects pharyngeal nerve plexus, throat, neck, nose, mouth, teeth, and ears
    - vibrates to the color sky blue
6. Brow:
    - located at the middle of the forehead (inside the head)
    - the place of intuition and soul knowledge; oversees the activities of the chakras below it
    - linked to hypothalamus and pituitary glands
    - effects nerves in head, brain, eyes, and face
    - vibrates to the color indigo or deep royal blue
7. Crown:
    - at the top of the head
    - the input center of spiritual energies, provides direct link to Source, and deals with all issues of spirituality
    - linked to the pineal gland (the body's light detector)

- affects the brain and the rest of the body
- vibrates to the color violet

The Usui Reiki Symbol and Attunements

As I mentioned in the preface, Usui Reiki symbols are considered sacred and are to be kept confidential. These symbols are important and very interesting in the practice of Reiki. They are simple words or phrases from Japanese or Sanskrit that help the practitioner to focus life-force energy during treatment. Life-force energy flows through all living things, and enhancing and focusing this energy with Reiki is the essence of treatment.

There are four basic Usui symbols taught to students of Reiki at different levels as they progress in their learning of this art. Students are asked to memorize the symbol and its meaning and application in the healing process. During the attunement, the energy of each symbol is imbued (brought down) to the students' minds and bodies. Once attuned to the energy of a symbol, the students retain this energy for a lifetime.

Other symbols are used by the master during the attunement. I discuss these more fully in the section about giving attunements. I am not enclosing photos of these symbols or divulging the words or phrases involved with each in this book, as it my belief that they should only be given to a student directly by a Master.

Please note: there are books and teachings that use other symbols and claim them to be Usui Reiki symbols, but they are not. Only the symbols passed down by those obtaining Mastership from Mrs. Takata or those of her direct lineage are considered authentic.

In addition, if a person is shown a Reiki symbol without the benefit of the attunement that empowers it, he or she may incorrectly believe that he or she has (the power of) Reiki and not take the class, thus missing the real experience of Reiki and losing the benefit of its healing power.

The Attunement

Healers may use life-force energy, or Ki, in the healing work they do, but not all use Reiki. Reiki is a special kind of life-force energy that can only be channeled by an individual who has been attuned to do so. As I mentioned earlier, Reiki is not taught the same way as other healing techniques, in that the Reiki Master transfers this special life-force energy to the student during the attunement process. Attunement is the only way to open the heart, crown, and palm chakras to that special link between the student and the Reiki source.

The Reiki attunement is a powerful spiritual experience. The process is guided through the Reiki Master by Rei or God-consciousness, to the student and automatically makes adjustments to the individual student's needs. As Reiki guides and spiritual beings are also in attendance at an attunement, many students have reported mystical experiences involving personal messages, healings, or visions. The attunement can also increase creativity, psychic sensitivities and perceptions, and enhance intuition.

Once attuned to a certain level of Reiki, it is yours for life. It does not wear off, and you never lose it. While only one attunement is required for each level, additional attunements may bring added benefit.

Reiki attunements can start as a cleansing process that affects the physical body as well as the mind and emotions. Toxins that have been stored in the body may be released, and thoughts and feelings that are no longer useful may be removed. It is recommended that the student be aware and conscious of this process and heed the signals of the body, mind, and emotions in the weeks after the attunement. Drink plenty of water, get outdoors often, breathe in healing oxygen, and get plenty of rest. You will feel great for it!!

The Power Symbol

The Power symbol is usually given to a student during training in Level One. It is used to "call in" and to increase the energy and power of the treatment. It is traditionally used at the beginning of a treatment and can be applied anytime during the treatment to enhance the energy as needed and in the end to seal the energies. It can be used to protect self, possessions, and those you hold dear. Because Reiki works on all levels—physical, mental, emotional, and spiritual—the Power symbol protects on all levels as well.

Prerequisites to the Healing Technique

A healing session or treatment involves calling in the spiritually-guided life-force energy of Reiki and transmitting it to a client through the palms of your hand. Your hands may be laid on a specific area of interest (e.g., where pain or dis-ease is manifested), but for a full Reiki session, the whole body is treated by placing your hands on or a few inches above the areas that relate to the seven major chakras. There are several procedures that need to be learned prior to doing a treatment.

Scanning

Once you have been attuned to Reiki, even at the first level, your chakras are opened to Reiki energy, allowing it to flow more easily. As well, the attunement increases your own intuitive powers and heightens your sensitivity to the psychic energy around you and to that of the clients you treat. Using the palms of your hands, you may then sense where the client needs Reiki energy.

After preparing yourself for a session, ask your Reiki guides to show you where imbalances occur. Place your dominant hand (the one you write with) over the client's body at a level of one to four inches, and starting from the head, slowly move your hand over the body in a downward smoothing motion. Let yourself be aware of what the palm of your hand feels. You may feel coolness or heat, a pulsing or tiny shock waves, pressure and tingling in one area and not another. You may find your hand pulled to a certain area. Just go with it, even if you think it is just your imagination. Make a mental note of the sensation and the area involved and move on. Or let your hand remain over the area until the flow of Reiki subsides. When doing the actual treatment, spend more time on the noted areas until you feel the balance occurring or that area feels the same as the area around it.

As you interact with the client's energy field, you will become intimately connected with him or her and aware of many things on a physical, emotional, mental, and spiritual level. Always honor a client's privacy and treat him or her with respect and dignity no matter what you may sense. Share this information with the client only if you are guided to do so and then always with kindness and respect, never with judgement or a lecture.

Reiki is sacred work! Always treat it as such.

Self-Scanning

To perform a scan on yourself, either kneel on the floor or lie down on a bed and follow the procedure as outlined above. You will need to ask for guidance and allow yourself to be open and nonjudgmental as you slowly scan over your own body and note any distortions you may feel. Allow yourself to feel any feeling that may be brought to your consciousness during this process. This is a very private process, as you are being made aware of deep physical, mental, emotional, and spiritual needs you may have. Treat yourself with the same kindness and respect you would a client. Be ready to forgive as necessary, and let the healing love-light flow in. This process will enhance your own sensitivity and promote personal growth.

Grounding

Chi, or life-force energy, animates and flows through all living beings. This energy is at once both positive and negative, as is all nature. Consider fire: it is a source of warmth and comfort, but it can be destructive as well depending upon the application or intent in its use. Chi or Ki is a non-physical energy used by healers. It is present all around us and can be accumulated and/or guided by intent. When working with this energy, it is recommended that you "ground" or "earth" yourself to form a complete circuit of the healing energy of Ki that connects your Higher Self, the client, and the earth. This practice helps the healing process by moving negative energy back to the earth and channelling in the healing energy. Grounding is accomplished by your intention to do so.

Exercises to aid the grounding process:

- Standing with your feet flat on the floor, place your hands together in prayer position above your head. Bring them down both sides of your body in a sweeping motion while visualizing the negative, excess, or no-longer-needed energy flowing downward. After you have finished the downward sweep, shake off your hands as though getting rid of something (water perhaps) while you imagine it dissipating into the earth.

- Standing or sitting with your feet flat on the floor, visualize a long, fluid rope or string attached from your feet to a boulder or tree root deep in the earth. Then visualize the energy you feel as negative flowing down this rope to the earth.

  Invigorating life-force energy may be absorbed from the earth via the same rope.

  When working with a client at the sole chakra, you can use either of these techniques to ground the client as well.

  Always wash your hands in running water after a healing session to remove any excess or what you feel to be negative energy.

Considerations

Things to remember when healing with Reiki, whether on others or yourself:

- Relax and allow yourself to merge with the Reiki consciousness. Once you have asked your Reiki guides for their assistance, trust that it is given.
- Hone your intuition. Let yourself be guided by what feels right. Follow your impressions, even if you think they are weird.
- Don't be attached to results, such as whether you are doing it correctly or not, or whether the person is healing or not. Remember that you cannot make a mistake with Reiki. The energy goes where it is needed.

- Do not push or force the energy. Simply relax and allow it to flow. Reiki *will* flow simply by your intent that it should do so.
- Be humble! You are not creating this. You are only a channel.
- Reiki is a blessing; use it as much as possible. Remember that the more Reiki you give, the stronger the flow of the Reiki energy will be within you.
- Also remember that all living things contain life-force energy. There is never a lack of it in the universe. My personal Reiki guide has given me a few simple exercises to help me understand this. I share these concepts, which my guide, Serus, calls Quatran later in this text, but following is a simple exercise to help you stay connected with the universal life-force energy.

Consider this corollary:

All living things on this planet require water for life. This is one of the most plentiful elements Mother Nature provides, and it flows freely for all. Water runs in rivers, is stored in lakes, and falls down as rain. Humans are, in fact, over 70 percent water in composition. You are part of it all and all is part of you. Do you see this?

Secondly, all animal life requires oxygen. All plant life requires carbon dioxide for photosynthesis (the food assimilation process) and exudes oxygen. Humans intake oxygen and expel the other gasses needed for plant life to grow. Do you see how much you are part of it all and all is part of you?

Connecting Exercise

Upon awakening, drink a full glass of water and consider how much water is part of you and part of all that is ... how it flows.

Now go outside (dressed for the weather!) and inhale deeply through the nose, and then exhale through the mouth, being consciously aware of taking in life-giving oxygen and exhaling carbon dioxide. Give the gift of your waste air to a plant or shrub nearby. It will thank you for it! Repeat this breathing exercise two more times, giving thanks to God as you know him for the bounty and abundance in your life this day.

The Healing Session: Pointers for Reiki Practitioners

1. Prepare the room prior to receiving a client. Soften the lighting, be sure the room is comfortably warm, play soft music, and perhaps use a scented candle or diffuser (though be sure these are acceptable to the client; ask if you don't know). Cleanse the room of unwanted energy. Using your whole hand, draw the Power symbol into the room, directing the energy of this symbol to the four walls, the ceiling, and the floor. Visualize healing energy filling the room.
2. Prepare yourself. Wash your hands, wear comfortable clothing, and remove watches and jewelery that may interfere with your work. Meditate or say a brief prayer for Reiki guidance, draw symbols into your palms, and say the sacred word or phrase three times. Ground yourself well.
3. Greet and establish a rapport with your client. Explain what you will be doing and invite him or her to be assertive about his or her needs as the treatment is given (as many treatments last close to an hour, the client may want to visit the washroom beforehand). Remind the client (and

yourself) of what he or she may experience, such as a release of tension, relaxation, hot or cold energy, tears, or jerking of muscles with relaxation. Honor the client's body's need and encourage relaxation. Ask him or her not to cross legs or arms, as this can interrupt the flow of energy.

4. Ask the client to remove shoes, watches, necklaces, and any restricting clothing, such as a tight belt. Make sure the client is lying down, with pillows placed for comfort, and covered with an afghan or soft blanket. Make sure that you are comfortably standing or seated during the treatment or you may become fatigued. Do not cross your legs.

5. If the client has a pacemaker or hearing aid, do not work over it but around the area. For clients who have diabetes, begin by working the sole chakra. If the client has had injury, pain, or surgery, work that area for a longer period of time.

6. Keeping the fingers together affords a stronger treatment. Keep your hands over each of the major chakras and any pertinent area for about three minutes while giving a Reiki treatment. If you move too quickly, the energy contact will be superficial. For the most effective treatment, use a very light touch of your hands on the body or a few inches above it. Keep your hand within the client's energy field, or aura, at all times as you move from place to place during the treatment, so as not to interrupt the energy flow. The energy field will extend an inch or more outside the client's body. You will come to feel it as you work with the client.

7. Always remember that you are working within a client's aura and personal space, so defer to him or her at all times. Some

areas (such as the genital or base area) are often very private or painful, so extra care should be taken here. However, these areas should not be missed or skipped in treatment, as all chakras are part of the whole. Placing the hands a few inches above or near the area may be more comfortable for both of you.

8. Do not diagnose but encourage the client to share what he or she has experienced and is feeling. Let your own intuitive powers and your Reiki guides guide you in the work. Reiki energy will go where it is needed, and the client's own natural healing systems will accept and receive as needed.
9. Seal the energy (as described below) after the treatment and thank your Reiki guides for assistance given. Release excess energy and wash your hands thoroughly after giving treatment.

The Healing Crisis

Although I do not like the phrase "healing crisis," it is universally recognized as the term used for the somewhat uncomfortable reactions that may occur after a healing treatment. When doing Reiki treatments and attunements, the client should be apprised of the possibility of some sort of reaction from the process.

As you know, Reiki treatments and attunements work to balance and realign the physical, mental, emotional, and spiritual body, assisting in the body's own natural healing process. This healing process may involve removal of toxins, ridding the self of unwanted habits, or facing hidden, unresolved emotions. All of these healing actions can cause some physical or emotional discomfort for the short term. If the client finds himself or herself running to the bathroom more often, or feeling weepy or sleepy, just gently let him or her know that this too will pass. Encourage the client to relax and recognize the benefits of the detoxification and release. If this is the first session with this client, be sure to follow up either with a phone call or another appointment within a week. Remind the client that, should he or she have any healing "symptoms," they are the body's natural way of ridding itself of unwanted and/or negative aspects. The client will feel much better for it.

Be aware that you too will notice activity and healing actions as you use this special healing art more and progress through the training. I tell my students that after an attunement, they will never be the same again. They will be better! And their journeys into healing and enlightenment will continue as they learn and practice more. This is one of the blessings of Reiki.

The Treatment

When using the spirit-guided life-force energy of Reiki to help heal yourself or others, you are drawing into yourself and transferring this wonderful energy. It should be your primary intent that healing takes place using Reiki energy to aid the body's own healing process. There are numerous ways of performing a treatment. In the Usui tradition, after you finish your preparations, you would typically begin the treatment at the crown chakra and work downward through all the chakras, ending at the feet for grounding. You should do a scan at some point to help pinpoint troubled areas. Let that energy flow and your hands go where needed. Trust your guidance and your intuition. The more you do Reiki, the more easily and more powerfully it flows.

The Procedure

1. Prepare the room as mentioned and cleanse it using the Power symbol as mentioned in Pointers for Reiki Practitioners, leaving the room filled with loving light energy.
2. Greet the client and ensure he or she is comfortably resting on the Reiki table. Ask the client to relax and close his or her eyes.
3. Prepare yourself. Stand behind the head of the table. Draw the sacred symbols into your hands and repeat the mantra associated with it three times, asking for assistance and guidance of spirit or your Reiki guides. Ensure you are standing comfortably and ground yourself well.
4. Touch the client lightly on the shoulders for rapport and ask if he or she is comfortable.
5. Begin the at the crown chakra by placing one hand at the crown and the other over the brow for a few minutes (unless the person is diabetic, in which case ground at the feet first and then return to the crown). For a full Reiki session, the hand should be held in all other positions for at least three minutes to reap full benefits.
6. Cup hands over the brow and eyes.
7. Place hands at each side of the face, and then at the base of the spine at the back of the neck, over the throat chakra, heart chakra, solar plexus, and sacral or base chakra. If you or your client is uncomfortable working over the base area, place your hands over the hips instead.
8. A scanning can be done at any time during the session. Run your left hand palm down over the major chakras from head

to base slowly. Allow yourself to feel and intuit what is there. Then work on the areas of concern a little longer.

9. Place your hands on both knees briefly, and then with a sweeping motion work down to the feet for grounding.
10. Hold a foot in each hand and ground well, mentally visualizing all unwanted energy being drawn down to Earth.
11. At this point, if you feel more work is needed, you may ask the client to turn on his or her stomach and work over each chakra again from crown to spine.
12. Rake off negative energies with a sweeping motion from crown to feet.
13. Close or seal the chakras in the zipper or close-the-flower ritual. (see page 21) This procedure is performed because often as the chakras are worked on, they open up to release things or to absorb healing light energy, but to leave them open may leave the client vulnerable. Alternatively, the body may have absorbed needed energies, and they should be sealed in. Reiki energy and the body energy intuitively know what is needed.
14. Place your client in a protective light by drawing an oval pattern around him or her with your hand and visualize the oval being filled with golden white or violet light.
15. Give thanks to your guides for their assistance. Shake off any unwanted energy with a chopping motion in front of yourself.
16. Allow the client to relax for a bit while you wash your hands thoroughly, and bring him or her a glass of water. Give the

client time to discuss the session if he or she chooses to do so.

Quick-Means Treatment

There may be times when you would like to give a full Reiki treatment, but circumstances don't allow it. At these times you can give a powerful Reiki healing session in an abbreviated form. This treatment technique is also applicable to self-healing.

After preparing the room and yourself, have your client sit in an upright chair in the center of an area where you can walk all the way around it. Ask the client to place his or her feet flat on the floor and arms at his or her side or comfortably resting on the lap. Be sure that your client is comfortable, and then ask him or her to close his or her eyes and relax.

After making contact with the client's energy field and at a distance comfortable to him or her, gently smooth the aura by moving downward from the top of the head.

Positions:

1. Gently place your hands on the client's shoulders for rapport.
2. Lay your hands briefly on the crown (7th chakra).
3. Lay your hands on the temples.
4. Lay one hand over the eyes and forehead and the other on the base of the skull (6th chakra).
5. Lay hand one hand over the throat and the other over the back of the neck (5th chakra).

6. Lay one hand over the chest and the other on the upper back (4th chakra).
7. Lay one hand over the solar plexus and the other in the middle of the back (3rd chakra).
8. Lay one hand on the abdomen two inches below the belly button and the other on the lower back (2nd chakra).
9. Lay one hand over the groin area and the other on the tailbone (1st chakra).
10. While supporting the client's leg with one hand or on your lap, place your hand on his or her knee and sweep down to the sole of the foot, placing your hand there for grounding. Do the same with the other leg and foot.
11. Complete the treatment with a brief soothing of the aura; close off the energy with a brief closing-the-flower, zipping-up-the-zipper, or any ritual you feel applicable to sealing the healing energy within the client and disconnecting from your energy source. Thank the Reiki guides for their presence with you.
12. Ask the client to breathe in deeply and slowly, exhale, and open his or her eyes. Remind your client of possible healing crisis after a treatment, especially if he or she has not been treated with Reiki before.

Closing the Chakras

Closing the Flower

Place your hands above the client or touch him or her lightly on the shoulders. Visualize the Reiki energy in the form of a flower, and then visualize the petals slowly closing over each chakra. Bless your client and thank the Reiki guides for their assistance and presence with you.

Zipping the Zipper

Visualize a zipper on the front of the body over the chakras. Beginning at the base chakra, zip it closed in a single smooth motion.

Self-Reiki

A Reiki self-treatment should be done daily, either upon awakening or before going to bed at night. This process should be undertaken for at least four weeks after the attunement. You can do this seated or lying down, though when doing a seated treatment you can more easily reach the back areas of each chakra.

1. Draw the Power symbol in the palm of your hand and do a scan of your body.
2. Place your hand over each chakra for a few minutes as shown in the Quick Means Treatment for Reiki. Rest the back of your hand over the areas you can't reach with your palms.
3. Feel the energy and visualize the color of each chakra as you work over it.
4. Close the chakras.
5. Upon completion of this process, give thanks to your Reiki guides and shake off any excess energy you may be feeling.
6. Relax and enjoy the treatment.
7. Practice, practice, practice.

— 2 —

Reiki Level Two

The Mental/Emotional Symbol

In Level One, I discussed the chakras and how Reiki assists the healing process on the physical level. In Level Two you will learn that the chakras also affect the mental and emotional levels of our being. Although all the Reiki symbols and mantras relate to the physical, mental, emotional, and spiritual aspects, certain symbols work more harmoniously with specific aspects. The Mental/Emotional symbol is one of these. This symbol used alone or with the Power symbol is especially effective in emotional and mental healing. It balances the right and left side of the brain and brings harmony and peace. It is especially useful when dealing with relationship problems and mental/emotional difficulties such as anger control, nervousness, and depression. Because of its harmonizing effect on the brain and emotions, this symbol is effective in healing addictions and improving memory. Also, the subconscious mind is more deeply affected when combining the Mental/Emotional symbol with your own affirmations. This symbol affords a special blessing to practitioner and client alike in its balancing and harmonizing of mind, emotions, and spirit. *Always use it (and all Reiki symbols) with love and honorable intent.*

In addition to the physical body, glandular systems, and nerve centers, the chakras also relate to, are affected by, and affect the mental and emotional parts of our being. Each chakra also responds to color, sound vibrations, and certain gemstones, aromas, herbs, and plants. The ancient healers used all of these resources to assist the body's own healing process. Whether it is used in conjunction with the Power symbol, with other healing aids like herbs or sounds, or on its own, the Mental/Emotional symbol is a very effective healing tool.

Chakras Reflecting Mental/Emotional

Just as each of the seven major chakras reflects to the physical body, they are also involved with the mental, emotional, and spiritual aspects of the living being. It is, therefore, helpful to learn and be aware of these aspects as you Reiki the chakras. The chart below reviews the chakra location, the color it vibrates to, and defines the mental, emotional, and spiritual aspect related to it.

Chakra	Color	Location	Definition
7	violet	crown	knowledge, spirituality, understanding, and universal consciousness *I know*
6	indigo	mid brow	intuition, future visions, dreams, abstract ideas, spiritual awareness, individual consciousness *I see*

5	blue	throat	memory concepts, the past, old habits and traditions, communication, expression, creativity, abundance, and receiving *I speak*
4	green	mid-chest	emotions, security, unconditional love, unity, relationships, affinity, giving, and receiving *I love*
3	yellow	solar plexus	intellect, mental awareness, self-respect, personal power and self-definition, will, and control *I can*
2	orange	navel area	social activity, belonging, acceptance, emotions, sensations, sexuality, appetite, pleasure, and movement *I feel*
1	red	base of the spine	the physical now, instinct, touch, foundation, survival, grounding, money, job, home *I have*

Healing Unwanted Habits

Few of us do not have habits that we find no longer serve us or may even harm us. Ridding yourself of unwanted habits (such as smoking, alcohol, drugs, being overweight, or anger issues) can be much more successful with the use of the mental/emotional Reiki symbol. A suggested method:

Be very clear about what it is you would like to eliminate or change. Write this down on a piece of paper along with your name and the Mental/Emotional symbol. Then hold the paper between your hands and Reiki it. This will send Reiki to the part of your mind and emotions involved with this habit. Do this for twenty minutes or more per day. Carry the paper with you, and when you feel an unwanted compulsion, take out the paper and Reiki it. It is not appropriate to do this for clients, but you may teach them how to do it for themselves.

Other Applications for Reiki

Reiki can be used in many aspects of your daily life. For example, Reiki can be used for cleansing a room of seemingly negative or unwanted energy, protecting vehicles and home or business, sending along with a gift or card, and treating plants.

Treating Plants

To Reiki a plant, draw the Power symbol in your hand and repeat the sacred name three times. Then project it toward the plant with love for a few minute each day. Thank the plant for being. You will be pleased with the results.

Treating Animals

Larger animals are treated like you would a client. Reiki the animal to the back of the head and down the spine, following the chakras. Be aware that a family pet or animal that is familiar with you and trusts you will be easier to work with. It will instinctively know when it has received enough Reiki and move away. Small dogs and cats respond well to just Reiki at the neck, behind the ears, or over the damaged area.

Protection

Draw the Power and Mental/Emotional symbols in your hand and say the sacred name three times. Project this energy into the room, home, car, or business you wish to protect. Alternatively, you may write the name of the area you want to protect on a paper and Reiki this paper. Trust the Reiki to do its work for you. To clear a room of unwanted or harmful energies or when preparing for a client, draw the Power symbol and/or the Mental/Emotional in your hand, repeating the sacred names three times. Project this energy to the four corners of the room as well as floor and ceiling. You may visualize the unwanted energies leaving the room via a door or window.

Sending Reiki

Gifts, cards, gems, and crystals may be given Reiki and sent to your loved ones with a healing/loving intent by holding them between your hands and drawing the symbols over them as you say the mantras for each. (This technique can be enhanced by the Distance symbol (see chapter 3) when you are attuned to it.)

Be creative. Use Reiki often in your daily life to protect, heal, and send love and healing light. Reiki is enhanced by use and never diminished.

— 3 —

Reiki Level Three

Distance Reiki

Like the first two symbols (the Power symbol and the Mental/Emotional symbol), the Distance symbol is transcendental in its function. The Distance Reiki symbol invokes the spiritual aspect of Reiki in that with your intent to send Reiki at a distance and your request for spiritual guidance to do so, the Reiki energy *is* transferred as requested. The power and effectiveness of this symbol comes from the attunement process and should be honored as sacred. This symbol is used to send Reiki to others at a distance, be it across the room, across town, or across the world. Neither distance nor time is a barrier when using this symbol. Use it to send healing love and light to a friend or loved one who is away, to send Reiki to the future when you know a specific time or date you feel you may need special care, or into the past to heal a traumatic experience you, a loved one, or a client encountered at a specific time in the past. When sending Reiki to someone at a distance, he or she should be aware of your intent to do so, either by the client's request or your suggestion of intent to do so.

The Process

Sending distance Reiki is a two-part process:

1. Establish contact using the person's name or a picture (or date and time specifics). When doing Reiki for the future (e.g., a surgery or dental appointment), note the time and date and be specific. When Reiki is done for past trauma, again, be as specific as possible about the incident, time, and date of the occurrence.
2. Ask for guidance, and then send the Reiki. There are several ways to accomplish this:
    a. Use a picture: draw the Distance symbol on the back with the name of the person, and then stand in front of the picture and beam Reiki to it.
    b. Do the above but then place the picture or information between your hands and request Reiki flow to the person or situation. This is particularly effective for time and situation healing.
    c. Draw the symbol into you palm and simply hold it in the direction you believe the person to be. Visualize the person with you as you send Reiki to each chakra.
    d. You may use a stand-in, like a teddy bear, and do a Quick Means Reiki on it on a person's behalf.

All of these methods are effective, as your intent, caring, and love are transmitted via your Reiki guides to the intended person at your request. Send Reiki to your personal spiritual mentor (God, Buddha, Jesus, personal angels, or guides) with your gratitude and blessing for the abundance and love given you. People have done this and reported receiving tremendous healing back from these spiritual beings.

Group Distance Healing

Distance healing can be sent by a group of Reiki practitioners with powerful results. This procedure can be done for a friend who is away, ill, or in danger; for a difficult world situation; to heal a communal trauma; or any number of situations that affect others. Here I describe two methods of doing this, but if you are creative, you may find others.

The Spiral

With the destination clear in their minds, each person stands facing the back of the one before him or her, sending Reiki to that person. The person in the front of the spiral beams the collective Reiki energy to the person or situation as agreed for a certain amount of time. The first person may then break away and move to the back of the spiral, allowing the next person in the line to beam out the energy.

The Circle

Each practitioner sits facing the center of a circle, sending Reiki to the center of the circle.

Procedure:

1. Be clear as to the purpose of the sending (to whom, to what situation, for how long).
2. Place a picture, word, or diagram depicting the person or situation in need of healing in front of the spiral or in the center of the circle.
3. Everyone draws the symbols and repeats the name of the symbol three times, and then the name of the person or

situation. Next, everyone beams Reiki out through the spiral or to the center of the circle to the to intended for a minimum of three minutes, meditating on the desired outcome.

4. Have someone do a brief benediction or closing at the end of the sending.

Empowering Goals

If you have been blocked in the achievement of certain goals or have not manifested the desired attributes as well as you would like, Reiki can help! Reiki energy is, after all, life-force energy and spirit-guided, so it brings a loving harmony into your life that can be directed to your own best interest.

Write your name on a piece of paper, and then write your goal and describe it as clearly as you can. Draw all three symbols—Power, Mental/Emotional, and Distance—on the paper. Send Reiki to this paper for at least twenty minutes per day. If this goal is in harmony with your highest and best good, you will achieve it! If it is not, you will find other ways to do what is best for you.

If the goal you seek is global (e.g., peace in the Middle East), proceed as above and know your love, prayer, positive thoughts, and healing touch do make a difference. You may find yourself presented with new ways to make this difference within your own sphere of influence, such as your home or community. Reiki is powerful!! Use it often.

Meditation

Because Reiki is spirit-guided life-force energy and involves the spiritual aspect of life, I have included a section on meditation. Learning to meditate, even briefly, on a daily basis can enhance Reiki power and your own intuitiveness to a greater degree. It will bring relaxation and serenity.

Meditation is the act of contemplation, of reflection, or of concentrating and directing one's thoughts on something specific or on nothing at all. It's also a way to empty one's mind for the purpose of relaxation or to achieve enlightenment.

The History of Meditation

Throughout history, mankind has shown an awareness of a Supreme Being or at least the knowledge that something greater and more powerful than the self exists. Examples of mankind's desire to find ways to connect with and appease this Supreme Being through rituals, sacrifice, prayer, and meditation abound in all different races and religions. There are many documented rituals from many different religions about the preparations made for meditation and prayer, such as facing in a specific direction (east toward Mecca), fasting, flogging of one's body, or doing a "walkabout." However, no matter what the ritual involved, the ultimate goal is to quiet one's mind and body for a time and just relax with one's highest self, God within, or the Supreme Being as the individual comprehends this Being to be.

Meditation is not a religion or faith, and in fact transcends all faiths and religions to become a personal act of relaxation and communication with the Supreme Being as that individual perceives this Being to be.

The rituals are just the human way of achieving the relaxation and desired concentration. Spirit is ever ready and simply waits.

Prayer and Meditation

Traditionally, prayer was considered to be "talking to God," and meditation was seen as "listening." Actually, both are forms of communication.

Meditation has three distinct sections. I call the first section "intent." Intent is where more than 80 percent of humanity spends its time when it decides to talk with God. It is received well by the Spirit, but it is only the "hello" portion of meditation. The second section is the process or stance, and the third is relaxing with the Spirit to listen and receive.

The Process

The ways people go about meditating are as varied as the people who perform the act. There are, however, several threads of similarity that run through all techniques.

Goal: the purpose of this exercise is to quiet your mind and body so as to allow the Spirit, God, or/and the Higher Self to communicate in real and subtle ways, and to allow yourself to open to these teachings and messages while the body and mind are fully relaxed but alert.

Meditation is not sleeping. Indeed, medical measurements of the brain activity of people who meditate and those who are asleep are very different. Also, vital signs such as respiration, blood pressure, and pulse are more relaxed and normal while a person meditates after he or she has learned to do so properly.

Intent: the desire to meditate for whatever the reason. Just reading this indicates a desire to, at the very least, learn about this process. Many people consciously make a pact with themselves to meditate at intervals that work for them.

Stance: meditation should be performed in a place that is quiet and away from disturbing noise and other stimulus. As the aim is to quiet the body as well as the mind, it is important to start by being as comfortable as possible.

Here are a few tips:

- Make sure the room in which you choose to meditate is not too brightly lit and that the temperature is comfortable for you. Meditating in a favorite spot outside on a warm day can be very relaxing. Playing soft music and lighting candles may add to the feeling of relaxation.
- Eat only a light meal before meditating; the body's natural process of digestion takes a lot of energy. Be sure you visit the toilet if necessary before beginning the process, as a full bladder can be very distracting!
- Wear loose, comfortable clothes and remove watches, belts, or anything that may distract you.
- Sit upright in a comfortable chair with your feet flat on the floor, your back straight, with your head perched comfortably on top of the spine. The idea is to have as few muscles as possible involved. Let your hands rest on the arms of the chair or your lap and let the chair take the weight of your body. It may help to imagine your spine as a string of beads on a beam of light. One end of thread of light holding the beads is connected to the sky (heavens) through to top of your head and grounded to earth at the base of the spine. Your vertebrae sit one on top of the other along this string of light. Your body rests comfortably along this string of vertebrae, held in place by muscle and bone.

A Relaxing Meditation

I will share one way in which I relax and let it flow. It involves some visualization or imagining, but I find it easier than just emptying the mind. Read this through all the way to the end of the meditation and then find a quiet place and time to try it.

Sit comfortably in your chair, back straight, feet flat on the floor. Let the chair hold your weight. Loosen any restricting clothing.

Take a deep breath through your nose; hold it a second and then exhale through your mouth. Repeat two more times, letting your body relax as you do so. Consciously listen to your breathing, without altering your breath, for a moment or two. Hear your heartbeat slow and easy as your body relaxes even more.

Now imagine yourself resting in a lounge chair on a deserted beach. It's just you, the waves gently splashing on the shore, the sun on your skin, and a gentle breeze. Feel the warmth of the sun, smell the ocean's scent, and hear the sound of the waves splashing on the shore. Let your mind and your senses immerse you in this scene. You are safe, you are comfortable, and you are caressed and loved.

As you relax here on the shore, a soft sound draws your attention. Maybe it's the soft call of a bird, or the wind rustling in the trees, but it draws your attention to the left along the shore. You notice a stand of trees and a pathway leading into them.

Relaxed but curious now, you find yourself going to the stand of trees and meandering along a sun-dappled path in the forest. Smell the pine, hear the faint call of a forest bird and the sigh of the wind in the treetops, and feel the warmth of the sun as it glints on the path among the trees. Sense the safety and the love of all creation around you. Immerse yourself into it and make this little forest grove your own haven as you walk along, sharing the joy of this place with the flowers, birds, animals, and trees. You are so very dearly loved here!

As you continue your journey, you come to a clearing in this magical forest with a small stone bench beneath a large oak tree. You skip over to the bench and sit down, watching the vibrant life of the world around you—the sun dancing on the grassy glade, a bird twittering, a brook or maybe a distant waterfall, and flowers in great abundance and in many colors.

As you sit here, you become aware of a special presence nearby that seems to call to you. Maybe it is a special flower, a bird, an animal, or a loving spirit. Identify it and claim this special being as your own by either going to it or calling it to you as you sit on the stone bench under the tree in the forest glade.

Communicate your appreciation and love, share your Big Question if you have one, and just sit there quietly for a few moments in the presence of this special being, accepting the love offered.

After a few moments say your goodbye, knowing that you can always return to this place and to this Presence at any time you choose, for you have just met your Higher Self, the God within, and she is there for you always, only a breath or a heartbeat away. Express your gratitude and thanks for this encounter, and wend your way back down the path to the beach and from there to the chair you are sitting on in your own home.

Take a few deep breaths, stretch, and have a large drink of water. You feel great! So relaxed, energized, and loved!

You can repeat this exercise many times and personalize it for yourself.

Remember that there are many ways to meditate. This is just one I personally find useful.

Moving Meditation

This form of meditation involves movement. I've compiled it from several disciplines, including yoga, Tai Chi, and Qui Gong, as well as from information received from an e-pal who runs Buddhist meditation seminars. The movements are very simple and should be done slowly to the count of three. Read this several times before beginning so you can follow without too many interruptions. I find this exercise to be most helpful when done first thing in the morning after the connecting exercise I described on page 14.

Movements:

1. Stand with your back straight and knees slightly bent. Visualize your spine as a slightly taut string of beads strung along a beam of light that travels from the Source through your head and down your spine.
2. Looking straight ahead, find a spot level with your eyes. Now move your head to the right, keeping your eyes moving horizontally at the same level. Hold for the count of three and then move it back to center.
3. Slowly do the same thing to the left to the count of three and back to center.
4. Look straight ahead and fixing on a spot directly in front of you, move your head down to the count of three, moving your eyes vertically in a line. Then move back to center.
5. Close your eyes and drop your ear down to your shoulder (do not bring your shoulder up) for the count of three and then move back to center. Repeat with your other ear.
6. Bring your shoulders up to your ears for a three-count and drop them back to normal.

7. Using the same slow three-count technique, do the following: raise arms above your head and then back down. Stretch your arms out to the side, level with your shoulder, and then back. Make a cradle with your arms and swing first right, then left several times moving your head along with the swing as though rocking a baby (in Qui Gong, this is known as rocking the baby dragon).
8. Bring your arms up above your head and then bring them down as far as you can toward the floor as you slowly bend from the waist, stretching the spine for a three-count and back to normal.
9. Standing relaxed, place your right foot out to the side so the instep touches the floor. Raise and lower your foot slightly to the count of three and bring it back. Repeat with left foot.
10. Stand straight, knees slightly bent and hands fisted at your waist. Now step forward with the left foot and bring your right arm up and down as though you had a sword in your hand and were slicing downward. Then bring the fist back to your waist (slaying the dragon). Repeat by stepping forward with the left foot and using the right arm as a sword arm. Release your fists and drop your hands to your side.
11. Stand straight, knees slightly bent, close your eyes, and step back with one foot. Bend back from the waist with your arms dangling at your side. Visualize your whole body grounding to Earth for a three count and then come back up. Open your eyes. Repeat with other foot and then open your eyes.

12. Sit comfortably in a chair and let your mind be totally blank for a few moments. If this is difficult, listen to your own breathing or heartbeat. If thoughts intrude, tell yourself that you will remember them later and relax.

Remember, no one is testing you on this! It is your own thing done your own way. Once you have mastered the moves and found the gentle three-count rhythm, you will find it enjoyable and relaxing and feel more centered and invigorated during your daily life.

Give thanks for the blessing received and go on with your day.

You have now completed the requirements to become a Reiki practitioner. Now its practice and more practice. The more you use Reiki, the more powerful the connection becomes, and daily meditation strengthens the inner healing and inner knowing as well. You may want to use this art only for yourself, your family, and a few friends, or you may want to set up your own Reiki practice and serve clients. Once you have confidence in your ability, you may want to teach others this wonderful healing art. The next chapters help prepare you for teaching Reiki.

— 4 —

Toward Becoming a Reiki Master

Working toward becoming a Reiki Master is a journey. It involves learning more about Reiki and becoming aware of what Reiki can accomplish in your life and the lives of others. It is a journey of discovery of the Spirit and your own understanding of the workings of the Spirit in and around you. It is journey of healing as well as self-discovery.

Thus far on your personal Reiki journey, you have learned about the history of this healing art, the chakras, how these chakras relate to the physical, emotional, and mental aspects of living, and how Reiki can balance and align these energy points. You have learned how to draw universal life-force energy to yourself using the Reiki Power symbol and how to direct it through your hands to yourself and others. You will have been attuned to this symbol, as well as the Mental/Emotional and Distance symbols, and have become proficient in using them in the traditional Usui treatment positions. By now you will be aware of how to use this healing love energy on yourself, plants, animals, and your fellow humans and how to use it for protection, cleansing, and to assist you in realizing your goals and aspirations.

Having learned the first levels of Reiki as taught by your Reiki Master, you are familiar with and practice the Reiki ideals and recognize the Reiki symbols as powerful and sacred. You are learning to trust your own inner knowledge and intuitiveness while giving treatments and practicing this wonderful art. Following the teachings and example of your Reiki Master, you are using professional etiquette while doing treatment, and you always regard any client information as personal and confidential. You treat your clients, fellow therapists, and yourself with respect, dignity, and care.

You may not yet have mastered all of the above concepts, but you have come a long way! If you feel you need clarification or practice regarding any of the topics I've covered, speak with your Reiki Master.

Overview of the Next Steps of the Journey

After a review, you will decide what it is that you need to learn more about or practice more. In this section I will answer commonly asked questions to the best of my ability.

1. We will discuss and practice meditation with Reiki; you will become more familiar with your personal Reiki guides and mentors.
2. I will guide you through a series of exercises designed for self-discovery and to help you to know where you are going from here.
3. Together we will build a Reiki Grid for Distance Reiki and empowerment.
4. You will discover the concept of, procedure for, and use of psychic surgery.

5. You will be given more Reiki symbols and learn the procedure for giving attunements to others.

Once attuned as a Master, you will be able to teach and attune others while continuing to learn and grow yourself.

Reiki Meditation

Find a quiet place so you will not be disturbed and just relax into the following:

1. Stand with your feet slightly apart and knees loose or sit up straight in a comfortable chair with your feet flat on the floor and hands resting on your lap. Lower your chin slightly and visualize a beam of light flowing from the top of your head, down your spine, and then down to the ground.
2. Draw the Reiki symbols you know in front of you using your whole hand to do so.
3. Raise your hands above your head. Feel the vibrations of energy and Reiki love light flush through you.
4. Bring your hands back down to the heart chakra and into the prayer position (*gassho*). Breathe in deeply and then expel the energy into your hand.
5. Now bring your hands to the brow chakra, visualizing and feeling the flow of indigo energy into the brow for a few minutes.
6. Move your hands down through the chakras, visualizing the color and feeling the energy of each chakra as you move down to base. Take your time. Feel the warmth, the love, and the flow of energy.

7. Now brush your hands down from your hips to your knees and then your feet. Ground yourself firmly to Mother Earth.
8. Bring your hands back up to the crown chakra in a single flowing motion (like closing a zipper) to close the chakras.
9. Give thanks to your Reiki guides for the blessings given.

Do this mediation daily for a while until you are comfortable with it and feel the flow, and then as often as you like. It is to your benefit to do so.

4

4 4

4

Quatran

Quatran is a concept and process of obtaining spiritual, physical, mental, and financial well-being. This concept uses the power of mentorship and angelic love. My Reiki spirit guide gave me this exercise. It is a concept to assist in self-awareness.

Individuals are offered this concept through a mentor. I have included this program in the Reiki Masters manual for students as a gift and a means of self-evaluation.

How well each succeeds is up to the individual. There are no tests here!

Mission Statement

It is our belief that:

The world can be changed for the better—one person at a time.

Our Earth provides bountifully for all—we just need to learn how to tap into that source.

The source of all power and abundance lies within the self.

We are not alone, we have never been alone. We are deeply loved.

At Quatran, it is our intent to assist you through the process of bringing spiritual, mental, physical, and financial well-being into your being.

Are you ready to make some changes in your life now, or are you just curious?

Good! Please continue to read this message.

What we ask of you:

1. That you accept the gift offered.
2. Confidentiality. A little bit of knowledge can be more dangerous than none at all, so we ask that you not share this concept or process (Quatran) with others until you have been attuned as a Reiki Master.
3. Four hours of your time per week until the process is finished.
4. That you use only environmentally-friendly products for yourself and in your personal environment (home, work, yard, etc.). Check with your Reiki Master if you are unsure.

Overview of the process:

1. Connect and familiarize
2. Cleanse and rebuild
3. Remove and reconstruct
4. Share and grow

How well you do in this process is judged only by you and depends only upon you.

You are deeply loved.

Quatran Contract

I, ________________________, agree to the following in acceptance of the Quatran mentorship concept:

- I accept the guidance and spiritual gifts offered.
- I will hold confidential all matters regarding the Quatran concept and process.
- I will set aside four hours per week to follow the instructions given.
- I will purchase and use only Earth-friendly products around my home and for myself where possible and choose a healthful lifestyle at least for the duration of this process.

Signature ________________________________ Date _______

Lesson 1

Planet Earth is a unique and wonderful place in the vast universes of God's creation. We of the angelic realm are honored to work with you here. We come only in love and in service to you. We have always been here for you. We are pure love energy weaving in, around, and through all that is. I am Serus. I come in love and service to you from a far galaxy you call the Dog Star. I am greatly honored to be a part of the Membership of the Family of Light from the other side of the veil, from a dimension other than your own, who are present on planet Earth at this time. I am mentor and guide to my Earth partner (Marguerite) and am presenting to you through her in service and in love.

We are not gods and would never, ever want to be deemed to be such, for we honor and love the same omnipotent, omnipresent God as you do. Nor do we come to take over your life for you, for this is not allowed by God! You, the human being on planet Earth, are marvelous and unique in the universes in that you are creatures of free will; you have freedom of choice that is given you by God and can never be taken away. Never, ever give away that freedom! Whether it is to a perceived god, another human, a habit, or a quest—do not give away your God-given freedom of choice.

You are part of the magnificent whole, as we are. We come, as I have said, in love and service to you.

My partner has set forth an exercise to help you grasp this concept (see the Connecting Exercise on page 13 in chapter 1). We suggest you review this again and practice it.

We would speak this day of money and your anxiety surrounding this and the issues of abundance. We, of the angelic realm, have no need for, nor do we worry ourselves about this, but we do understand your concerns. We say to you that planet Earth has provided for all and all may have access to this bounty! Not so, you say. But yes, this is so. Consider this. In the early stages of man's history upon Earth, humans were hunters and gatherers.

They took freely of what the earth had to offer. Using intuition, innate intelligence, and the lessons learned from their forbearers, they followed the wandering herds and gleaned from the earth that which they needed for survival. They also understood the seasons, the ebb and flow patterns inherent to the area in which they lived, and were able to store away some of their bounty for leaner times.

Money, we say, is merely energy, a commodity of exchange that humans have devised for trade and commerce. You, my dear ones, still have the same instincts, talents, and innate intelligence as your forefathers and Mother Earth provides. Worry not! Open to all the abundance available to you, choose wisely, and all will be well.

My partner has set forth a few lessons to help clarify this matter for you, should you choose to follow them.

Connecting Exercise: see (page 13) Chapter 1

Upon awakening, drink a full glass of water, being aware of how much water is part of you and part of all that is. How it flows.

Secondly, go outside (dressed for the weather!) and inhale deeply through the nose and exhale through the mouth, being consciously aware of taking in life-giving oxygen and expelling carbon dioxide. Give the gift of your waste air to a tree or shrub nearby. It will thank you for it. Do this three times and then give thanks to God, as you know Him, for the bounty of this day and for the angelic presence in your life now.

Worksheet 1: Clarification

Find or buy an empty notebook.

Date all pages as you proceed.

On the first page, top and center, draw the Quatran logo. Then draw the Reiki Power symbol (to bring in the great beaming light) in the center of the page.

On the inside leaf of the first page, write a short paragraph outlining your expectations of the Quatran process as you understand it now.

On the last page of the book, draw a vertical line down the center. On the left, outline any physical problems you may be having today, and on the right any mental or/and emotional concerns.

On the two second-from-last pages, draw horizontal lines through the center of each page. Remember to date the pages.

Top left: enter the family income expected this month and give a percentage as to what your income is and that of your partner (if applicable). Be as accurate as you can.

Top right: give a dollar value to all the essentials for life for yourself and family. Be honest about what is really essential (e.g., food, shelter, medication, fuel, and transportation to work).

Bottom left: give a dollar value to all debts owed and the amount of the monthly payments.

Bottom right: write a dollar value of all last month's actual expenses categorized in groups (e.g., food, shelter, etc.).

Do this as accurately as you can. This is simply for your own clarification. Close the book.

Do the Reiki meditation as taught. Feel the vibrations of Reiki light flush though you to release all tension and relax your mind, body, and spirit. You are one with all that is.

Lesson 2

I am Serus, come to you with love and in service. You, my dear ones, are dearly loved. We have said we are with you always and we are. Know this. We are here but do not interfere, coming only when called. This is the great and wonderful part of your being human—an animate, corporal being and a spark of the Divine. You, unique in the universes, have been given freedom of choice. What a marvel you are! We are honored to work and interact with you.

The young (and not so young) have asked, "Why am I here now? What is my purpose?" We say you are here on Earth at this time by choice, and your purpose is to be, *to have being and aliveness. Your physical body is a vehicle, if you will, for this journey you are on. And yes, dear one, it is a journey and an adventure every day. Do you understand how wonderful your biology is? Cherish this physical body you have and the environment in which you now live. As a piece of God, a spark of light on Earth, you have been given a place to be that supports you in every way, and the tools and talents to live this life in joy and happiness as you travel your own pathway. We do not interfere but watch with great delight and anticipation. We are but a heartbeat away, waiting for your conscious awareness of us and what we offer.*

"So what can I do?" you ask. Begin, we say, by taking heed of the physical—your body and intimate environment. Do you see how magnificent the human body is, how when it functions well, all that is good follows? Do you yet comprehend how the environment in which you choose to live enhances your whole being? Think well on these things!

Of late, in the now, your bodies and intimate environment have been challenged. This is not to be feared, merely brought to your awareness. Pollution, be it mental, physical, electromagnetic, or emotional, is the antithesis to your well-being. Be aware of this and listen to biology. Take steps to protect yourself from these now.

You are dearly loved and very important to the whole even as you live now. You have great work to do. We would wish that that you remain on Earth for a very, very long time, dear ones.

Take care of yourself first. *A cleansing of self and your environment will bring increased good health, well-being, and clarity.*

My partner has set forth a few duties for you to follow for the enhancement of the physical body and your intimate environment. Should you choose to follow these instructions, you will be well rewarded in kind.

You are dearly loved. Serus.

Worksheet 2: Cleanse

1. Remove all home and self-cleaning products that are not environmentally safe and place them in a box. Replace with environmentally safe products, like tea tree oils, evergreen products, or hydrogen peroxide in lieu of bleach. Also, remove all vitamins and supplements that are not tested for safety. Check with the pharmacy or your Reiki Master if you're not sure. Do this for at least for the duration of this exercise.
2. Thoroughly clean your home, car, and other living areas with these safe products as directed. Pay special attention to rugs, furniture, drapes, and other areas that are not cleaned as regularly and to heating ducts and furnace filters. A few drops of tea tree oil, citronella, or lavender oil on the filter will help to cleanse the air. Remove and throw out vacuum bags often, and if you have a lot of insects in your home, try a mothball in the vacuum bag. It smells for a bit but will help remove insects and larvae. This is not to imply that your home is dirty or you are a poor housekeeper. I am merely trying to draw your attention to and aid in cleansing the environment in which you live.
3. If you do not do so already, consciously drink more clean water. It helps to flush impurities from your system. Add a natural source multivitamin to your daily regimen and an antioxidant. Continue this for at least three months.
4. Choose an exercise routine that suits your goals and lifestyle, and practice it faithfully for a few months before you adjudge the results.

5. Rid your home, vehicle, and workplace of extraneous *stuff.* Give away and recycle everything you no longer need.
6. Continue the Connecting Exercise and take a moment in the evening for prayer or meditation to give thanks to God as you know Him for the blessing of that day.

Open your notebook to the last page. Have the physical concerns you had gone away or abated after completing the above exercise? If not, have you formulated a plan or concept to help your body/mind/spirit heal? You can discuss this with your Reiki Master if you like.

On the second-from-the-front page, date it and list at least four talents you have and at least four positive characteristics you possess.

Now write down some of the things you like about your home, your workplace, your environment, and the town (city) in which you live.

On the next page, date it and write down what you deem to be the blessings in your life (physical, mental, people, places, etc.). Just let it flow.

Close your notebook.

Do the Reiki meditation from page 42.

Open your body to cleanse at the cellular level and accept an infusion of Reiki light. Feel it flow.

Lesson 3

I am Serus, coming to you in service and with love. You, dear one, are to be congratulated and are greatly honored for the work done in lessons 1 and 2. You have accomplished much, have you not? Honor yourself for this, dear one. And continue to live your life path as you, long ago, chose it. Yes—you chose it; we merely assist and aid at your calling and your wish. You are greatly honored and loved. Know this!

We would like to repeat again, as you take your journey, to **take care of yourself first**.

As we watch and observe the interrelations between you humans, we have a fine chuckle—not at your expense, but with you. Ah! The little dramas you create amongst yourselves. We ponder this and realize that you have not yet understood that these are no longer necessary. You are a piece of God on Earth in lesson, but you no longer need these little interrelational dramas to learn those lessons. You, the enlightened ones, can now learn by directly accessing the part of God within, by observing and honing your intuitive powers, and finding ways to make every incident a win-win situation for all concerned.

You know this. You remember. Yes, you do!

All those little hurts you feel are caused by others in your life who you are desperately trying to please and appease, to gain their respect, but it is all to no avail, isn't it? Did not your Great Teacher say to you, "Love your neighbor as you love yourself." Do you get it? "As yourself." As you remember who you are (a piece of God on Earth) and love yourself for it, all else falls into place. Yes, this is so. And you will chuckle with us over all the small stuff that has given you such pain. Yes, you will.

So what are the dramas of which we speak? The small dishonesty of your mate, the one-upmanship you play at work, the hurts you allow yourself to feel when a loved one doesn't intuitively sense what you want or need. Even the mind games you play with yourself about what you want to do and/

or have accomplished are dramas. You know the ones. Stop this and look around you. Is your life not good, even great? So why do you waste time with these games? What purpose do they serve? Ask yourself that. What is it that you need of Spirit, of yourself, that requires you to play out these dramas? Learn the answer from within. "Ask and it shall be given you, seek and you shall find" are familiar words, aren't they? Apply these ideals to your relationships and talk with your loved ones, coworkers, and friends. Talk and listen, listen, listen, and listen. The way to a win–win situation will become abundantly clear.

Always remember, dear one, you do not necessarily know what is best for another, only for yourself! That is how it is. It is in taking care of yourself with honesty and true intent that the best for all will follow.

I am becoming preachy here (my partner says) so I will not belabor this point further, except to wish for you the highest and best. For that is what you are.

My partner will outline a few tasks to assist you in this. If you choose to do them and do them with integrity, you will be well rewarded.

You are dearly loved and highly honored. Serus.

Worksheet 3:

Open your notebook to the last page. Have the problems you mentioned there abated or lessened? If not, make note and discuss it with your Reiki Master. Have you found a financial future that looks brighter now, less worrisome?

Take time to evaluate the concepts and process of Quatran as you know it so far.

Go to the next page in the back of your notebook and date it. Mark down the names of all the people in your life now and evaluate them as L (loved one), F (friend), or A (acquaintance). Write these names quickly and evaluate them clearly as you go.

What are your expectations of each type of relationship (e.g., what do you expect of a friend)? List these expectations.

What are your responsibilities to each type? Write them down. If you have questions, ask your Reiki Master.

Close your notebook book.

Think well on this lesson with prayer and meditation. Take time to let the concept "gel."

Open the notebook to the next front page and date it. Write down the blessings you have received from each group.

Close your notebook once more.

In doing this process, you will find that some people in your life do not currently provide you with anything of value or seem to drain your energy. Understand that these may not be the best relationships for you, and that this is fine. Some folks pass through our lives for just an instant and all they and we need is provided in that instant. Others stay a little longer but are not meant to be permanent fixtures in our lives. Learning to let go of relationships that no longer serve your highest interest is as difficult as working to keep a relationship alive. Sometimes it is best to let go, and sometimes the effort needed in keeping the relationship alive is worth it. Only you can judge what is best for yourself. According to the teachings of Serus, a dead relationship will die gracefully when no more energy is put into it, and there is no fault in this. And a worthy relationship will also die when it is not energized. It is the natural way.

Keep your home, vehicle, and workplace clean and free of unnecessary clutter. Reuse, sell, or recycle what you can.

Continue to do the connecting exercise in lesson 1 and keep yourself and your environment physically and spiritually clean.

Daily meditation is an asset here. Treat yourself to this pleasure often. You have now completed Quatran.

You may want to keep your notebook for reference and add new ideas and concepts that help you build your enlightened life.

Although Serus has not dictated a fourth lesson per se, many of his missives to me have been about sharing the concept of Reiki and other energy healing arts, as well as growing in our own personal spiritual lives. It is my understanding, from his missives, that it is now a very opportune time for humans to learn, share, and grow in spirit and in harmony with one another. Other spirit-guide works, like Kryon, channeled by Lee Carroll; Archangel Michael, channeled by Celia Fenn; or Veronica, channeled by April Crawford speak of this as well. Check it out!

Having completed the Quatran series, ask yourself:

1. What have I learned about myself regarding the physical, mental, emotional, spiritual, and financial aspects of my life? Do I see areas that need improvement, and do I see clearly the way to improve? Do I recognize that I am much more, much better, much more capable than I thought I was? Give thanks for this. Recognize that you are changing and growing continually and that you can do so with elegance and grace.
2. Is meditation becoming more comfortable? Am I more aware of the Spirit working within me as I Reiki myself and others? What do I recognize as the Spirit (Reiki energy) enters? A feeling of warmth, lightness in the air around me, a gentle stroke on the forehead? Let yourself feel these moments, and learn to recognize this and more.

The Reiki Grid

Sylvia Browne, Lee Carroll, Greg Braden, and other "seers" of our modern world recognize the increased momentum of the mass awakening of individuals to a higher consciousness. They recognize how Spirit is at work in the world today as more and more people, who they call "lightworkers," are learning to use this energy and apply it to the betterment of self and mankind. These seers also recognize, as the ancients did, the value of using crystals to anchor the limitless universal life-force energy.

When setting up a Reiki grid, you must be fully aware that for Reiki to work, you must intend that it do so. Simply put, you must intend for the Reiki energy flow to ensure that it does.

Quartz crystals have the unique property of being able to absorb and hold thought and intentions. Therefore, these are the crystals that are most often used in Reiki grids, though other conductive stones like amethyst, jade, and rose quartz may also be used. There are many texts written about the use of gemstones in healing. Choose stones that "speak" to you or use a pendulum to aid your choice. To make a Reiki grid, you will need eight crystals—six for the outside that are slightly pointed and five to eight inches long, one longer pointed one to be used as the Master Crystal, and a center stone. The center stone may be quartz or any other conductive stone and may be a cluster, a ball, or a pyramid.

After obtaining the eight crystals for the grid, you must cleanse them of any impure or inappropriate energy that may be clinging to them. This can be done in several ways. You can place the stones in a bowl of rocks or sea salt. Make sure they are totally covered, and then ask that these stones be cleansed and blessed with your intent to use them on a Reiki grid. Leave them for twenty-four hours. Or you may leave them in direct sunlight or moonlight with the same intent for twenty-four hours. Then remove them and place them in a paper or wooden container or in a natural cloth bag until you are ready to use them on the grid.

The Reiki grid is a hexagram (six-sided figure), also known as the Antahkarana symbol to those who know yoga. A copy of this figure will be given you by your Reiki Master or you may copy it from the resources sited at the back of this book.

Place the hexagram on a stiff cardboard or wooden tray. On the back of a picture of yourself or on a page with your name on it, write that you affirm your desire to heal with love and wisdom. Place this affirmation under the center of the grid.

Charge the crystals you will be using by placing them in your hands and drawing the Power and Distance symbols over them, visualizing the energy empowering each crystal. Speak a prayer of meditation over each, expressing your desire that the original Reiki Master or your guide bless them with your intent to heal yourself and others with this grid. Place the six crystals at the six corners of the hexagram with the pointed side toward the center of the grid. Now put the center stone over the center and your picture.

Take the Master Crystal in your hands and Reiki it with the Power, Master, and any other symbols you may feel you need at this time. Hold it in your hand until you feel the energy warm and vibrate. Now use this Master Crystal to charge the grid as follows.

Move the Master Crystal over an outer stone, down to center, and up to the same stone again. Moving clockwise, do the same to each stone until you have worked over all the outer stones. Take your time. Move around the outer stones in this manner in a continuous motion at least eight times. As you do this, repeat your affirmations in a continuous refrain as well. Your affirmations may be something like, "I now charge this grid with light, with light, with light, to heal, to heal, to heal, I charge this grid with Reiki, with Reiki, with Reiki." Once charged with Reiki, the outer stones may be fixed to the paper with a small amount of glue, leaving the center and Master stones free. The grid is now ready to be used for specific healing, to send continuous Reiki to you or others, or to specific situations. It can be used to assist you in special goals or for ongoing inspiration. Simply place the name or request under the center stone over your picture and charge the grid with Reiki and your intent in the matter. You may recharge the grid daily or as you are guided to do by the Spirit.

As you become more comfortable with this method of using Reiki energy, you will find many ways to apply it for yourself, others, and different situations. Do not be afraid to experiment; just be sure to clearly indicate your intent, respectfully request the aid of Reiki guides or/and your own personal guides, and let it flow. Always remember to give thanks for the blessing given.

Psychic Surgery

Most people are not the best they can be physically, mentally, and/or emotionally at all times. Some never achieve their highest form, though all have the capacity to do so. This is because we humans allow, attract, or create blockages in the flow of life-force energy. These blockages usually result from ideas, beliefs, and/or emotions that are contrary to our own optimum well-being and can manifest symptoms that are physical, emotional, or mental in nature. Once these blockages are identified and released, the normal, natural flow of energy will return.

A technique called psychic surgery can be used to release these blockages.

First determine that the client feels he or she has an issue. *This is not for you to determine.* The client must state that he or she needs assistance with a specific issue, illness, or problem. You may explain what you do, but the client must determine the issue. Then you may ask the client to define it more definitively.

1. Ask the client to close his or her eyes and think about the problem.
2. Ask leading questions to help the client with this process, such as:
    - If the problem manifested in a body part, where in the body would it be?
    - What shape would it take—round, square, triangular?
    - What color is this shape, and what is its texture—lumpy, smooth, or rough?

- If the issue (problem) could translate into sound, what would this sound be?
- How does it taste or smell?

3. Let the client take time to formulate this picture.
4. When the client has a definite picture in his or her mind, ask if he or she is willing to let it go completely. Explain to the client that in this process, you will assist him or her in sending this issue to God, their Higher Power, Mother Earth, or whatever is comfortable to the client.

The Process

After determining the issue, have the client comfortably seated or laying on the Reiki table. This process may be performed along with the healing session as you usually do it or as a separate procedure. Ask the client to close his or her eyes and relax quietly as you prepare yourself.

Standing behind the client, draw the Master symbol in your hand three times, quietly repeat the name of the symbol, and then clap your hands together three times. Do the same with the Power symbol, and then draw it down your body for protection and draw smaller Power symbols over each of the major chakras on your body.

Extend the fingers of your Reiki hand and pull the fingers with your other hand as though you were pulling taffy, extending the pull to twelve to eighteen inches beyond your fingers. Draw a Power symbol over the extended fingers. Do the same with the other hand. This preparation doesn't take long but requires your full attention, focus, and concentration.

Be completely confident that your guides will be able to work with your clear intent to heal and that Reiki spirit-guided life-force energy is all-powerful.

Now place your hands on the client and ask him or her to think about and again describe the issue or problem in detail. As the client remains quietly relaxed, close your eyes, and with full intent and concentration, let your hands move to where they are needed.

Then, saying a pray for guidance, draw out the problem and ask that it be replaced with love energy. When drawing out the offending energy, make an audible sucking sound as you inhale and a gentle blowing, directed down to Mother Earth, as you exhale.

Do not take on this energy. Visualize it coming out of the client into a shape (like a ball) in your hand and then throw it to Earth or to the light. Repeat this process five to eight times, or as many times as you and the client feel is needed. Step away from the client with a downward stroke like a karate chop and shake off any excess energy. Ground yourself well. Draw the symbols into your palms again, and then step back to the client and draw a circle of healing love light around them. Give thanks to your guides for the assistance given.

Discuss with the client how he or she is now feeling. If the issue seems to be persistent, repeat the process at a later date. Remind the client of a possible healing crisis as a result of your work together and advise him or her to drink plenty of water, have a mild diet, and go out into the sunlight a lot in the next few days.

If the client's problem still does not dissipate after a few sessions, it may be that there is a lesson that needs to be learned. Meditation and prayerful attention to the client's own inner knowing will help to identify the lesson and assist in learning it with elegance and grace.

This technique works. It is a powerful tool to add to your healing repertoire.

Giving Attunements

Once you have been attuned as a Reiki Master, you may, in turn, attune other Reiki students. This process is a privilege and an honor and is to be approached with dignity and respect at all times. The attunement is an integral part of becoming a Reiki practitioner. It opens the heart, crown, and palm chakras to that special link between the student and Reiki source.

There are four parts to the process of giving an attunement:

1. opening of the crown chakra to bring Reiki energy into the aura
2. planting this energy into the hands, body, and chakras
3. sealing the connection between the student and Reiki source
4. Blessing the student and giving thanks for the gifts given.

There are several things a Reiki Master needs to know and practice before giving an attunement. He or she must:

a. be familiar with and able to draw the Tibetan Master symbol, the Usui Master symbol, and the Raku (thunderbolt or serpent of fire).

b. be able to hold contract and hold the Hui Yin for the duration of the attunement. Hui Yin is the practice of contracting the transverse perinea and pubococcygeus muscles around the anus and vagina in women and the anal muscle in men. At the same time as these muscles are contracted, you must hold your tongue to the roof of your mouth. This hold is done to retain the Reiki energy within the *hara* during the attunement. The *hara* is the area within the human energy field where we hold our intent.

"Beneath the human energy field lays the haric level, in which we hold our intentions. Our intentions have a tremendous importance in the creative process."—Barbara Ann Brennan, *Light Emerging*

The center of the haric level lies within the area of the sacral or second chakra.

c. be able to bring in the Violet Breath. While holding the Hui Yin, draw a breath and imagine white light flowing through your crown chakra and through your tongue, and then down the front of your body through the hara and up the back to form a cloud or mist within your head. Now imagine this mist rotating clockwise (unless otherwise directed by your guides) from the left ear over the top of the head to the right ear and around. Quickly allow this mist to turn from white to blue to violet. As this mist continues to rotate in your head, picture the Tibetan Master symbol within the mist in the center of your head. The symbol is stationary within the rotating mist of violet.

With practice, the Hui Yin and Violet Breath can be achieved quickly and easily. It is all in the intent.

Prepare the room and yourself for the attunement.

The room used for the attunement should be comfortable and free of noise or interference. You may place a single candle on a table in front of the student for focus and burn a scented candle if the student is comfortable with this. Cleanse the room with the Power symbol, as taught, on the ceiling, floor, and the four corners of the room. Say a prayer for guidance and help, and then draw the Usui and Tibetan Master and Power symbols into your hand, repeating their sacred names. Draw the Power symbol down your body and over each chakra.

Ensure that the student is comfortably seated in a straight-backed chair in an area of the room where you can move around him or her easily. Have the student close his or her eyes. Explain what will be occurring during the attunement and ask the student to relax and meditate or think positive thoughts as he or she places his or her hands in prayer position with the thumbs against the heart chakra. Remind the student that you will be moving his or her hands during the process.

Step 1. While standing behind the student, obtain energetic rapport. Ask silently that you be allowed into the student's energy field with a brief touch on the shoulder. Using your whole hand, draw the Raku or Serpent of Fire symbol down the student's back from head to hip and then three Usui Power symbols at the base.

Now place your hands on or directly over the student's head and holding the Hui Yin, form the Violet Light on your head. Hold the Hui Yin and your tongue to the roof of your mouth throughout the rest of the attunement. Gently blow the Violet Light into the crown and to the base of the brain. Then draw the Usui Master symbol over the head and direct it to the base of the brain along with the symbols you are *not* attuning the student with at this time (see chart on page 70).

Step 2. Bring the student's hands up to the top of the head, open the hands, and with your forefinger draw the appropriate symbol(s)—the one(s) they are being attuned to—into the open palms three times and tap lightly to implant. Close the hands and return them to the prayer position.

Step 3. Step to the front of the student, take his or her closed hands in yours, open them, and draw and implant the symbol(s) as in step 2. Close the hands, return them to prayer position, and gently blow Violet Light over the hands, down to the base, and back up to the heart chakra.

Step 4. Step behind the student again, look down into the root chakra from the crown, and visualize a bright red ball of light at the root. Say a prayer of guidance and affirmation for the student, and then seal the attunement with a Power symbol to the neck area.

Step 5. Stand a little in front of the student with your palms open toward him or her and send a blessing and the Violet Light. Release the Hui Yin.

Step 6. Have the newly attuned student open his or her eyes and remain quiet for a moment to absorb what has just occurred. Suggest the student go outside for a deep breath of fresh air. Discuss what he or she may need to ask or express, and remind the student of a possible healing crisis as a result of the work you have done together today and how to deal with it. Let the student know you will be available should he or she need to call you.

Below is a chart of the symbols to be placed in the student's hand when giving the attunement.

Level 1: Power symbol

Level 2: Power and Mental/Emotional symbol

Level 3: Power, Mental/Emotional, and the Distance symbol

Master Teacher: all of the above as well as Tibetan Master, Usui Master, and Raku symbols

As Reiki Master, you now have the skills and knowledge to teach others. Remember, you are on a journey along with your students. It is a very personal journey, and as you open to Reiki energy and spirit, more and more is available to you.

May your journey bring you much joy, and may your lessons be learned with elegance and grace.

Appendix: Meeting Your Reiki Guide

As you become more aware of the life-force energy of Reiki thrumming through you, you will be opening more to the Spirit. Some of you may have already experienced some of the wonderful attributes of working with spirit-guided energy, such as a deeper sense of well-being, warmth in your hands and body as you work, meaningful dreams, or a gentle, feathery touch on your head or brow in meditation. You may want to be more familiar with your own personal Reiki guide or invite another Significant Being in to be your guide. Remember that though Reiki is not a specific faith, religion, or cult, it is spiritual. You may use a religious icon or angelic presence (e.g., Christ, Buddha) as your guide if you so choose.

Meeting Your Reiki Guide

Sit in a meditative position in a quiet place. Take a deep breath and relax.

1. Choose an enlightened being you'd like as your guide or simply be open and ask your spirit guide to come into your consciousness.

2. Get a picture of the enlightened being your wish to be your guide, or simply write his or her name on a piece of paper, or ask for conscious awareness.
3. Sit in a comfortable chair, draw the Reiki symbol on your hands, and give yourself Reiki for a few minutes.
4. Using your whole hand, draw the Distance symbol in the air in front of you.
5. Point your palms upward and make this affirmation: "I now send Reiki energy directly to (state the enlightened being's name or simply say "my guide") to create a strong energetic connection with him (or her) and ask him (or her) to be my spiritual guide(s)."
6. Then begin sending Distance Reiki to this being.
7. Continue doing this for at least fifteen minutes.
8. Occasionally repeat the affirmation during this time.
9. Give thanks for the connection that is developing.
10. Practice this meditation with reverence once a day. Be consciously aware and alert for any and all messages you may receive in your thoughts, dreams, daydreams, or in the natural world around you.

References

Andrews, Ted. *Animal Speak*. Woodbury, MN: Llewellyn Publications, 2000.

Brennan, Barbara Ann. *Light Emerging*. New York, NY: Bantam, 1993.

Brennan, Barbara Ann. *Hands of Light*. New York, NY: Bantam, 1988.

Lake, Medicine Grizzlybear. *Native Healer*. Wheaton, IL: Quest Books, 1992.

Rand, William L. *Registered Karuna Reiki Master Training Manual,* 2001 The International Center for Reiki Training, Southfield,MI

While writing this book, I drew upon information from classes taken with Lady Dr. D. Marshall at the International Academy of Natural Health Sciences and information given to me orally by Reiki Masters Shirley Ross and Ann Maynor. The Canadian Reiki Association (www.reiki.ca) and the International Center for Reiki Training (www.reiki.org) also provide valuable information in their newsletter and magazine on an ongoing basis.

Resources

The following are places to find further information about Reiki and to search for a Reiki Master should you desire to continue learning about this marvellous healing art:

The International Center for Reiki Training

William Lee Rand and his team of Lightworkers have provided books, seminars, a magazine, and a website (www.reiki.org). There is an information page that lists where the seminars are being held and as well as a list of Reiki Masters.

The Canadian Reiki Association

The website www.reiki.ca provides valuable information and a list of seminars and Reiki Masters available in Canada. This organization provides an interesting newsletter to keep you up to date on the latest happenings and offers a place to advertise your own local Reiki business.

— Notes —